EMERALD PUBLISHING

Explaining Alzheimer's and Dementia: More than Memories.

David Moore

www.emeraldpublishing.co.uk

Straightforward Guides
Brighton BN2 4EG

ISBN 9781847161703

Printed by GN Digital Books Essex

Cover design by Straightforward Graphics

About the Author

David Moore lives in West Sussex with his wife and two daughters.

Currently he is a training and development officer working for the Adults' Services training department, of West Sussex County Council.

David's background is in Mental Health, working with People with dementia. He has managed a number of services specifically for people with dementia including one of the first services for younger people in the UK. David worked for Dementia Care Matters Ltd for four years before becoming the chief assessor for EDIs VRQ in dementia care. David has a BSc and MSc in Health Psychology and is a qualified Dementia Care Mapper.

David has written a number of books about living with dementia including:

Guide to dementia care.
Building on strengths.
Making each day count.
Positive dementia care.
Understanding dementia.
Certificate in dementia care.

Dedication

For Kirsty, Daisy and Amber-Marie. I love you all so much .xxx

And

Grandad for the happy times we had together on Barmouth beach.

Acknowledgements

The *HOPE of people with experience* group including Les and Audrey Pepper, Christine and Willem Vandervalk, Graham Browne, Bob and Marilyn Noble and Jill Vigus.

The dedicated staff and customers of West Sussex County Council Adults' Services in particular Kirsty Jones, James Hodge, Dawn Budden, Marcus Batterbury, Jane Monday, Debbie Ryan, Allison Anderson and Shelagh Doonan.

Lisa Moulding, Julie Moulding and the staff, clients and relatives at Avon Manor – Worthing, West Sussex.

Simon Kral, Deputy manager of Glebelands Day Centre

Liz Bassett Manger and Shelia Talbot (deputy manager) of Maidenbower day centre.

Andrea Linell. Independent Consultant

Naresh Mapara and the staff and residents at Wykeham House Care Home, Surrey.

David McLaughlan and the staff and residents at Westergate House Care Home, West Sussex.

Julie Foster, Alzheimer's society – Horsham branch.

Donna Harwood and her staff and clients at Fernbank Care Home, West Sussex.

Pam Grey – Time out for Carers – Guild Care.

Anne Fretwell and Martin Lunn Merevale House, Atherstone, Warwickshire.

David Sheard, Peter Priednieks and Pat Kite of Dementia Care Matters Ltd.

Elayne Dunn, Cognitive Help and Therapy (CHAT) – Horsham.

Thank you for your words and advice that appear throughout this book.

Illustrated by Kirsty Moore

Clipart from www.freeclipartnow.com

Contents

Foreword

Since the introduction of the National Dementia Strategy for England in 2009, there seems to have been a increased acknowledgement of the difficulties people living with dementia can experience. However, the focus still seems to be on the disease and the negative image of dementia depicted by many. This book tries to rebalance the reality of living well with dementia.

I often reflect on my visits to see my Step-Grandad, Horace. His eyes would light up when he saw me and a big smile would fill his face. This was how he would always react to seeing me, the only difference now was due to his Alzheimer's he couldn't quite remember my name or who I was.

Despite his failing short-term memory there was still a connection between us, an unspoken understanding that being together brought us both happiness.

I'm sure we can all relate to this type of emotional connection. Have you ever met someone for the first time and although you don't yet know them, have made an instant decision on how they make you feel?

David explains in this book, through his own experience of working with people with dementia and the experiences of people he has met, that it is crucial we focus on the person with dementia as a person who has and still is travelling the journey of life who has the ability to feel emotions and connect with the world around them and ultimately to continue to live a fulfilling life.

Our being is not just based on our brain's capacity to remember and store information but on our ability to feel emotion, hence the title of this book, "More than memories".

Kirsty Jones
Older People's Mental Health Training and Development Team
West Sussex County Council.

Chapter One

"Have I had lunch yet?"

"Have I had lunch yet"? This simple question was one of the first key signs that not all was quite right with my Grandad. It was a question that would change my family's life forever. Over the coming years he and the rest of my family followed a path that many people in this country have had to take. A journey that incorporates many difficult battles. Facing up to the reality that something is not 'quite right', desperately trying to receive a diagnosis and then beginning the difficult job of learning how to live with it, in some cases without much support from the 'experts'.

I know there were times during my Grandad's illness that were incredibly hard for him and those who loved him. He felt great frustration at not knowing where his wife was, only to be reduced to tears by well meaning family members who reminded him that she had passed away many years ago.

My Grandad was never told his diagnosis. We all knew and yet when he begged us to tell him what was wrong, we told him it was just part of getting old. The first great difficulty to overcome was moving in with my family. This was incredibly challenging for a man who up until now had always had a 'quiet life', to suddenly be faced with trying to fit into the chaos of a busy household. After living with us for two years my Grandad moved into a care home, for all of us it felt as if we had betrayed him. We had promised him time and time again that we would never 'put him in a home' and yet here we found ourselves doing exactly that.

Feelings of guilt.

The family's feelings of guilt were not helped by the fact that we shortly had to move Grandad again as the original choice of care home could not cope with his 'challenging behaviour'.

Luckily the second care home was amazing. It felt like a 'home' rather then a hotel or a hospital. The staff treated my Grandad like 'Jim' not just another number or patient. He made good friends with the care staff and the other people with dementia who lived there. They encouraged him to regain lost skills and soon he was walking independently to church, something he had not done for many years.

My Grandad lived at the home for a number of years. We were lucky enough to visit him regularly and even though he would not remember my name he would always greet me with a smile.

Sadly he became ill and had to go into hospital. After only a few days of being in hospital he was given medication to 'calm him down'. We were told that the medication was needed because my Grandad would not stay in his bed and would walk around the ward.

The nature of the ward meant that the staff were very busy and simply did not have the time to support my Grandad, in the manner I am sure they would have liked to.

Darkest days.

My Grandad's darkest days were his last. Since his arrival on the ward, in a matter of a few weeks, we witnessed a massive change for the worse in him. I remember sitting there watching him, a withered and tired man who no longer wanted to live.

None of us had expected a 'happy ending' but none of us predicted an ending to my Grandad's life like that, lying in a hospital bed.

I have always questioned was it my Grandad's dementia that had caused him to decline so rapidly or was it his 'treatment' in hospital? I know the staff in the hospital were under terrible pressure and from speaking to people in preparation for this book things don't seem to have changed.

We have been working faster and faster with fewer staff. Its never been quite this Dickensian.

Staff are being asked to reapply for their own job.

At certain hospitals there are just not enough staff to do the job
.
Quotes from hospital staff.

The second care home had shown to me that living with dementia did not have to be the 'hell' that so many of us imagine it to be. The home had shown that life with dementia can still be one worth living IF the person with dementia and their family are given the right support, understanding and empathy. It taught me that it is possible to find direction and purpose with time and support from the right people. However my Grandad's experience in hospital also taught me that if this support is not there then a person's experience of dementia can be a dark one.

The big D

I have to be honest I didn't want to know the truth. I would have preferred to hear the doctor say anything......anything but that.

You can understand with the negative attitudes out there why people don't come out and say they've got dementia.

Quotes from Family members

I recently sat with a friend, whose mother had been diagnosed with dementia. She told me that, although deep down she knew that her mum had the illness, she had feared hearing the word dementia.

My friend is not alone. Dementia is probably the condition that more then any of us fear, the news that someone we care for or we ourselves have been diagnosed with this condition. It used to be the BIG C but now the BIG D seems to have truly taken the throne of the thing we fear most.

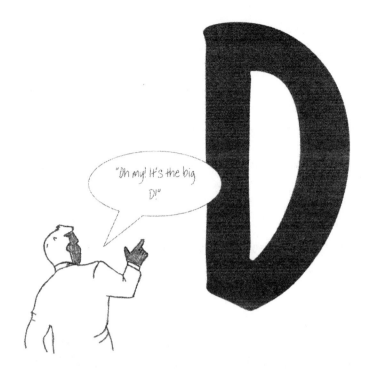

The big D.

During this conversation, with my friend, I asked her what she was going to do? She screamed the answer back at me that: *"she didn't have a clue"?*

Too often I have heard similar statements coming from numerous people:

- What do I do next?

- Who can help?

- How can I cope with this?

- Why did it happen to her/ him?

These are the kind of questions that too many people face and often there is no magic wand that can be used to give the answers.

The aim of this book is to at least try and start answering some of the questions people living with dementia may have. This book also aims to illustrate that, although living with dementia may seem the worst thing in the world, there is still hope, there is still a future to be shared and new goals can still be achieved IF we as a society recognise that people with dementia and their carers have a very valuable part to play in our society.

Don't ignore me. I'm still human and that's it in a nutshell.

Quote from a Person with dementia.

Being positive where possible. People out there think that dementia is all negative where as actually you have got to live for today.

Quote from Family carer.

The message, that has come across from many people with dementia, is that there are ways of living with dementia and the difficulties and challenges it can bring. This is different for each person. For some it can be through laughter, working with others, sharing their experiences with others, art, exercise, the company of good friends or religion.

The doctor said to me this morning I've got to cut down on the unhealthy food I am eating. She said fish is good. I said what with batter? I don't think she was impressed.

Laughter gets you through it.

I haven't got a broken arm or a plaster cast. I might go round with a bit of plaster on my head with the words dementia written on it.

I have fewer friends now but those who are left are good true friends.

My stepdaughter is one of those who thinks there is nothing wrong with me because I do talks up in London. Whereas my son knows more then me. He rings me three times a week to see what I am doing. My other daughter has never spoken about it she does not want to know. But I met her on Thursday at Eastbourne and we spent half a day together. She'd got a laptop for Christmas. When we sat there the other day she said you are on 'you tube' – it was three or four talks that I had done about having dementia. This is the first time since 2006 when I was diagnosed that she has sat down and spoken to me about my illness.

Quotes from People with dementia.

The next chapter of this book considers the different perspectives of dementia including the medical model and person centred care. It also reasons that the domination of the medical model can actually create an added burden to the person with dementia and those who support them.

One so called professional said to me, 'I suppose I won't get much information out of him?' I was livid.

Quote from a Care home manager.

My mother comes in and treats my husband as an exhibit. She peers around the door at him and then comes and talks to me.

Quote from a Family carer.

The third chapter discusses the significance of recongising a person's remaining strengths and abilities that can survive even into the later experience of dementia. This is in order to provide a wider view of what it is like to have dementia. The medical model often focuses on the losses and growing dependencies and ignores the importance of considering what a person can still do.

Chapter four aims to provide useful information about what dementia is and the different causes of dementia.

The fifth chapter explores how people use behaviour as a form of communication.

Chapter Six discusses the importance of being a good listener. This is so essential for people with dementia, to be shown that what they are saying is of value and importance. This chapter also indicates that although the language used by people with dementia may become harder to understand there is still meaning behind what people say or do.

Finally at the end of the book there are some useful contact details including the Alzheimer's Society.

****

Chapter Two

Different Views About Dementia.

This chapter considers some of the various views that are held about dementia.

The first part of the chapter looks at the dominant approach, known as the medical model, and how this has influenced professionals, the Medias and societies perception of what it is like to have dementia.

The second part of this chapter considers how there is an alternative way of thinking about dementia, known as person centred care. (The 'new culture of dementia care'). The underlying principle of this is that a person with dementia is a person first and foremost. This view recognises people with dementia are individuals who need understanding and support throughout their journey of dementia.

An added burden?

A family member once described to me the added burden the picture painted by the medical world brought to her caring role. When I asked her to explain what she meant by this she told me that everything she read or everyone she spoke to had told her to expect a future where her husband would become increasingly difficult and dependent. Yet she explained that this was not the case. She admitted there were times when things were *'damn hard'*, when she felt she could no longer cope and eventually her husband moved into a care home. However she also added they were some of the happiest times they had spent together. She told me that if she had been given a more *'balanced view'* about the future she probably would have felt more positive and consequently better prepared for living with dementia.

Of course I have bad days but I don't feel too bad today.

Bringing a bit of humour into our situation is fundamental because if you can't laugh about things you can't get through.

Quotes from People with dementia.

The question has to be asked surely a more balanced view of what living with dementia is like, both for the person and the carer, needs to be presented? However currently there seems to be one model that dominates and thus moulds the beliefs of many about what dementia is. This model is known as the medical model.

What is the medical model?

This approach focuses on the biological damage that occurs to the

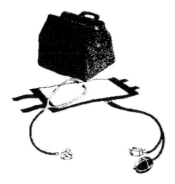

brain caused by the dementia and the resulting symptoms and behaviours. Yet, because of the medical models desire to find a cure and treatment for dementia, it has been criticised for concentrating too heavily on the 'science' of dementia and not exploring the individuality of each person with dementia.

This failure to consider the value of individuality means the focus has centered on the loss and pain dementia brings. Furthermore the model has led to the development of a fabricated belief that the journey of dementia is travelled solely by the carer, while the person with dementia become a shell of their former self, a 'living shell' a 'living death'.

The authority the medical model has can be seen in the limited number of people with dementia who are told their diagnosis. According to a report by the National Audit Office (1) very few people with dementia or their families are ever given their diagnosis, unlike in other European countries. (Current estimates are that in only about 30% of cases is a diagnosis given).

The decision not to give a person the **choice** whether to know their diagnosis or not may be based on certain professionals' *perception* about *dementia* and not on their knowledge about *the person*. They may believe that people with dementia will not be able to cope with the reality or will simply forget or not understand. This is the case for some people with dementia but certainly not all.

I've still not been told if it is dementia or not.

The doctors haven't said its dementia but she doesn't recongise us anymore.

Quotes from Family Carers

Because of my diagnosis she can ask me the questions she needs to why we've still got time left. When my mum and dad died twenty odd years ago I sat there thinking I never did ask them that question, I never did say sorry for that. Where as because I've had my diagnosis me and my daughter can talk.

I know what's wrong. I've always known what's wrong even if they won't tell me.

Quotes from People with dementia

For those people who could understand their diagnosis, being left in the dark will add to feelings of paranoia and will prevent a person being offered choices about support and treatment, such as counselling, links to a local Alzheimer's Society branch or a support group, being able to resolve financial matters and discuss with others the future before it is too late. So the reality is a person's choice to know is taken out of their hands, and consequently reflects treatment of people with cancer thirty-years ago. The person is forgotten in favour of the illness.

Despite the medical model being criticised for its failure to focus on the uniqueness of each person with dementia, it sill pervades many people's attitudes and beliefs about dementia.

My Grandad was telling people in the hospital that he had met the pope. They all thought he was mad but he had. He was a journalist and had met all these famous people including John Paul II.
Down in the hospital it's just like "him in bed number 3". They just seem to drag them out of bed.

Quotes from Family carers

One social worker came to visit me and she said to me 'I don't know much about your condition'. I couldn't believe what I was hearing.

I said to them what did you expect people with dementia to be like? They said they expected it to be people sitting in chairs around the wall. They were quite surprised to see it wasn't like that.

At one meeting one of the women was a manager and she didn't realise that people with dementia could live on their own. It is frightening when you have these people and they don't understand.

Quotes from People with dementia

I said to the hospital staff her name is Winifred but she likes to be called Jane but they still kept calling her Winifred.

Quote from a Manager of a care home

The medical model, has in turn, shaped the media's view of what it is like to live with dementia.

Media description

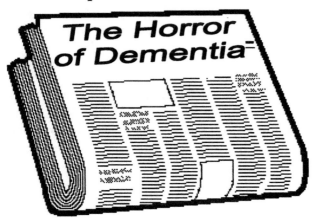

The papers use those headings to get people to look at it.

Basically they classed me as dead before they gave me a chance.

Quotes from People with dementia

The current stuff on TV reinforces the preconceptions rather then moving it forward to 'these are the difficulties but this is how you can manage it'.

Quote from a family carer

The media often focuses on the 'horror' of living with dementia. Often soaps and dramas depict the person with dementia as a 'crazy old person'! The following extract from a magazine highlights the image of trauma that can be portrayed.

"One look at the mass of scrambled nerves in a human brain afflicted by Alzheimer's disease is all you need to understand why sufferers are reduced to mumbling, fumbling, frightened shells of their former selves. No one could hope to retain their sanity with a mind that resembles a plate of spaghetti". (2)

This extract is not uncommon. Newspapers, magazines and books suggest a destitute image through the use of the language they use to describe dementia. Words such as sufferer, burden and demented are used as ways of describing people with dementia. Yet these words provide us with a very limited view of what it is like to experience dementia.

I don't consider myself to be a sufferer.

Quotes from a Person with dementia.

It is true that some people with dementia may suffer and may feel a burden, but there will be times when a person with dementia will feel happy and useful. However using the term *sufferer* gives the opinion that people are constantly suffering. This is not the case for a lot of people. Also the term evokes sympathy, feeling sorry for the person, something that may not be beneficial. Instead a person may benefit from empathy, trying to understand what the person is going through, walking in their shoes.

The media's portrayal of dementia has in turn greatly influenced society's view of what it is like to have dementia.

There is still this expectation that you hear the word dementia and there's a picture in people's minds of someone sat in a corner unable to communicate and dribbling. People were shocked that he looked normal and could communicate.

It comes back to that term dementia. The picture in your mind is someone who is at the end stage and is having to be cared for 24/ 7. Not the fact that there is a huge run in, years of independent, semi-independent living.

We don't use the word dementia. You can see people's shutters coming down. They glaze over and switch off. If you say memory problems that's fine they can relate to memory problems

I'm going to see my mother she is 92. She does not want my husband (who has dementia) to come along. Out of sight out of mind that's her view.

There is this whole stigma thing.

Young people with a family, as a general rule, families don't really want to get involved with the older generation.

Going from two daughters who were very understanding and sharing if you like.... we've only seen them once since Christmas.

Quotes from Family Carers

I hate it when some visitors come to the home. You can see them looking at the residents as if their going to be sick.

One of our residents had a visitor. I took her a cup of tea and biscuits and she asked me if we had different biscuits for the visitors. I told her that we all had the same biscuits.

The paper version of the person seems to have become more important than the one with the heart beat...when the inspectors come they want to look at the care plan rather than the person.
Quotes from Care home managers

I've been very hurt by things in my family, how they have reacted to my dementia.
Quote from a Person with dementia.

Baroness Warnock

Recently Baroness Warnock added fuel to the fire by declaring,

"If you are demented you are wasting people's lives, and you are wasting NHS resources".

Her views seem to represent the beliefs of those whose ideas are routed in care that has stemmed from the medical model of dementia.

There can be no denying that living with dementia is probably the biggest challenge any of us will have to face in our lives. Dementia can bring with it a great sense of loss and pain, both for the person living with the dementia and for those who know and support the person. But to believe that if you have dementia you are a waste, surely this view could never help anyone living with dementia? However things are changing......

Changing times, changing views?

Over the past twenty years growing numbers of inspirational husbands, wives, sons and daughters have openly challenged the traditional medical view of dementia.
Everybody's story is different.

Let's just talk about people.

We are with dementia where we were with cancer 30 years ago and that was known as the big C. Gradually those negative perceptions have been broken down and we can do the same with dementia.

Quotes from Family carers.

They have argued that there is no set journey or experience of caring for someone with dementia and that everyone will have a very **different** and **unique** journey of dementia. They have presented a more *'balanced view'* that illustrates not only the difficulties faced but also the hope and joy that can still be experienced

Many family members have openly discussed their experiences of living with dementia, both good and bad. People such as Barbra Pointoin, who allowed TV cameras into her life to film the journey she had supporting her husband Malcolm. Cora Phillips and Morella Kayman, who established the Alzheimer's Society , Ray Smith who described looking after his wife as the happiest time of his life (3) and Andrea Giles who wrote about the difficulties of caring for her mother in law (4).

When he first got his diagnosis I did phone them up (the GP surgery) and ask where do I go for help luckily they told me about the Alzheimer's society.

We did the best we could.

It changed everything. All I could feel was anger and I had no one to direct it at.

I've had to fight tooth and nail to get him a second day at the day centre.

You can't come across as reasoned, calm and collected or else they don't think there is a problem. You have to be tearing your hair out before anything is done.

I work with patients with dementia as well as having a husband with dementia.

It's never ending. You need to be problem solving constantly. You don't know what you need in the future until you need it. It's thinking on your feet!

I am expected to do half a dozen things at once.

We live in parallel words.

Quotes from Family members.

More recently people with dementia have been taking the platform to tell others about their experiences. Individuals such as the author Terry Practchet, Christine Bryden (5), Charles Schneider (6) and Peter Ashley have actively campaigned, written books, spoken at conferences, and developed online communities (7) to raise awareness about what it is like to live with dementia.

People with dementia have become involved in national and local projects such as the Alzheimer's society's living with dementia programme (8), West Sussex County Councils HOPE of people with experience group(9), and DeNDRoN (the Dementias and Neurodegenerative Diseases Research Network) (10).

People often say to me, ' I never would have guessed'. I don't have a flag on top of my head saying I've got dementia.

I went to do a talk for the Department of Health and they showed the new dementia advert that has been on the telly and a bloke asked me what I thought of it. I told him I thought it was rubbish because they have a white screen at the back that's saying that the person with dementia is blank, show them that they have got a life, show them working in the garden, with friends, down the pub. Show that people with dementia still have a life.

Just because I have got this thing doesn't mean its time to give up.

I can't show you what it is like...I wish I could.

I feel for my carer rather then myself. I think it is more difficult for her to cope with me. I can cope with what I am doing most of the time. My wife is lumbered with me all of the time, which I find very disconcerting. I don't think its fair that she's in this position but I can't do anything about it.

Quotes from People with dementia

These incredible individuals are challenging societies perception about what it is like to live with dementia.

Professionals who have challenged the medical model.

Also many forward thinking professionals have promoted the importance of creating a new culture that focuses on the person rather than the dementia. Most notably Professor Tom Kitwood, who was based at the University of Bradford, who applied the concept of person centred care to the field of dementia. This has been called the 'new culture of care'. Being person centred is about recognising that a person with dementia is a person first and foremost. They may have dementia but this is only one of the many factors that need to be considered when supporting them. Kitwood believed that all people with dementia should be valued and not treated like second-class citizens. He strongly argued that if people with dementia are given the opportunity to grow in confidence and feel good about themselves then this will help them cope through the journey of their illness.

Other professionals who have revolutionised the way we think of dementia include John Killick who has worked with people with dementia to publish their poetry and has set up the *'Dementia Positive'* website and Professor John Zeisel who has promoted the idea of *"the gift of Alzheimer's"*. Zeisel recognises that no one would wish for this illness however living with dementia can help us to refocus on what it means to be truly human and to appreciate the time we have been given.

I much prefer working with people with Alzheimer's than other jobs. You gain more rewards.
Working with families and people with dementia inspired me to become a nurse.

This is the best job I've ever had.
Quotes from Staff.

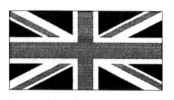

This crescendo of voices finally led to the British government publishing a five-year strategy to improve dementia care in England in 2009. The title of the strategy, *"Living well with dementia"*, shows that having the label of dementia is not a death sentence.
The people, who I have spoken to while researching this book, have shown me this. It is clear that having a chronic illness such as dementia can be incredibly difficult. It can be physically and mentally exhausting for the person with dementia and for those who care for them. But with the right support and understanding people with dementia and their carers can still have a life that can be full of good times.

The National Dementia Strategy has seventeen objectives to enable people to live well with dementia.
O1. Improving public and professional awareness and understanding.
O2. Good-quality early diagnosis and intervention for all.

O3. Good quality information for those diagnosed with dementia and their carers.

O4. Enabling easy access to care, support and advice following diagnosis.

O5. Development of structured peer support and learning networks.

O6. Improved community personal support services.

O7. Implementing the Carers' Strategy for people with dementia.

O8. Improved quality of care for dementia in general hospitals.

O9. Improved intermediate care for people with dementia.

O10. Housing support, related services and telecare.

O11. Living well with dementia in care homes.

O12. Improved end of life care for people with dementia.

O13. An informed and effective workforce for people with dementia.

O14. A joint commissioning strategy for dementia.

O15. Improved assessment and regulation of health and care services and how systems are working for people with dementia and their carers.

O16. A clear picture of research evidence and needs.

O17. Effective national and regional support for implementation of the strategy.

The National Dementia Strategy. Department of Health (2009).

Hopefully if you are a person with dementia reading this chapter it will have shown you that, despite all the challenges having dementia will throw at you and your family, you can still lead a fulfilling life.

If you support someone with dementia then the hope is that this chapter has shown you that there are two sides to every tale. There is no denying living with dementia is tough but it can be made a lot easier with the right support, right care and by working with the person you are caring for.

Five years ago when I gave up work to care for my husband my children were really supportive.

Quote from a family carer.

For all of us we need to consider how best to meet this challenge that our society faces. It's no use burying our heads in the sand hoping that everything will be OK. So the question we face is, do we embrace the medical models limited view or do we recognise that if the **right support** is provided people can **live well** with dementia?

(1) The National Audit Office (2007) Improving services and support for people with dementia
(2) Sainsbury's magazine 1996.
(3) Ray Smith (2004) Amazing Grace: Enjoying Alzheimer's. Metro Books, London.
(4) Andrea Gillies (2010) Keeper. Short Books. UK
(5) Christine Bryden (2005) "Dancing with Dementia - My Story of Living Positively with Dementia" Jessica Kingsley Publishers.
(6) Charles Schneider (2006) "Don't Bury Me...IT AIN'T OVER YET" Author House Publishers.
(7) DASN International is an Internet based support network organised by and for people with dementia. http://www.dasninternational.org/

(8) Living with Dementia, Alzheimer's Society, Devon House, 58 St Katharine's Way, London E1W 1JX

(9) HOPE of people with experience are a group of people with dementia who have been trained to facilitate training to health and social care professionals.

(10) DeNDRoN coordinating Centre, Wolfson Centre, Mecklenburgh Square, LONDON. WC1N 2AP.
http://www.dendron.org.uk/

The next chapter continues the theme of considering the alternative approach to the medical model. So chapter three will focus on people with dementias strengths and abilities first before moving on to considering what dementia is.

****

Chapter Three

Focus on strengths!

Its all about holding on to what the person still has....not letting go.

Quote from a Family member.

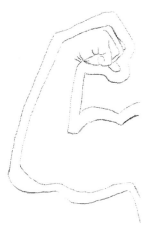

Chapter two discussed the important changes that have taken place in the perception of what it is like to live with dementia over the last twenty years.

The focus has moved from solely looking at people's dependencies and difficulties to an understanding of people's remaining abilities, in other words what people with dementia can still do.

It is clear that people with dementia will face losses and it is understandable that many people will focus on any deterioration because this seems to illustrate that the person with dementia is moving further away from the person they once were. However, people with dementia will also retain numerous skills and so this chapter considers some of those common abilities.

Graham.

A short time ago I met a gentlemen with dementia called Graham. We soon found that we had a common love for football and by chance his team had recently beaten my team. (7 -1). I thought to myself he wouldn't be able to remember the game however Graham soon started to take me through a detailed discussion of this game and others. This incident made me realise how often I still focus on the 'dementia' first before seeing the person. In other words because I knew Graham had dementia I presumed he wouldn't remember. It also made me consider how often we focus on a presumption of what a person with dementia won't be able to do rather then starting from the opposite end of the spectrum i.e. what can people still do. But you might ask why does this matter?

I believe that if we only concentrate on a person's losses this will ultimately have a detrimental effect on the self-esteem of the person with dementia and also our own belief of what a person can do. If we take over from people and do tasks that a person can still do independently, or with some encouragement, then not only will we cause the person frustration and embarrassment, we will also increase the chance of the person becoming more dependent on us. Finally, by focusing on skills rather then just losses, this is a way of helping people living with dementia to remain positive.

People are constantly reminding you that there is something wrong with you by highlighting what cock ups you've made.

When you start talking you know they are looking at you

thinking there's nothing wrong with him. It's because you can talk and you can be blunt and honest.

Quotes from People with Dementia

They asked us our views and then they totally ignored what we said. Why did they bother to ask us.....its just so they can tick a box. If there is a reason why something's not be done it would be nice be told why our advice was not listened to.

Quote from a Family Carer.

Some of the skills many people with dementia retain or develop include the ability to:

- Connect to music and song
- Appreciate Art
- Live for the moment
- Recall of Long term Memories
- Connect with emotions.
- Connect with others.
- Stay active.

The rest of the chapter will look at these abilities in turn.

An important role.

It is worth considering how people without dementia can support people with dementia to maintain these strengths. The reality is if people with dementia are not given the support or opportunity to maintain these skills then these may also be lost. Not because of the 'dementia' but because we have not enabled the person to maintain their existing abilities.

The ability to connect to music and song

Lizzy is often in her own world, but as soon as I start to sing to her a smile appears on her face.

The place where I worked we did music and stuff and it was all Max Bygraves. But interestingly the music that was the biggest hit was Abba.

Quotes from care staff.

There is now a vast amount of literature that looks at people with dementia and their ability to connect and find meaning in music. It is possible that music unlocks a person's memories. Melody, tone, rhythm and song are areas of the brain that seem to remain relatively untouched from the advance of dementia. There are many examples of where music is being used to connect and enhance the lives of people with dementia. For example the UK charity Live Music Now runs a scheme called *"Active Music, Active Minds"*, which promotes live music for people with dementia who are in care homes or hospitals across the country.

I have lost count of the number of times people have said to me they are amazed that a person with dementia they know struggles to produce a couple of words and yet when they hear a familiar song they can sing along.
Quote from a Manager of a care home

The ability to Appreciate Art

Art is being identified increasingly as being key.

Quote from a Family carer.

I go and do my drawings.

It passes the time of day beautifully. All you need is a pencil and rubber and away you go.

Quotes from people with dementia.

Art often gives people with dementia an opportunity to express their thoughts and feelings. I have been amazed about the number of people with dementia who I come across who have maintained a skill or found a new joy in art, whether it be painting, sculpture, poetry, carpentry or simply observing others creating art.

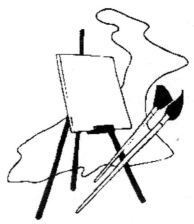

The ability to live for the moment

Some people with dementia have described how having dementia has enabled them to appreciate the moment.

After a few months (of having my diagnosis) I decided to book a holiday. It was the best decision I made.

Quote from a Person with dementia.

She didn't have a terrible quality of life. In fact she lived it to the full.

Quote from a Family member.

Throughout our lives we are often so busy worrying about the past or planning the future we often fail to consider what is happening in the moment and the positive things that are occurring. Often these are the simple things such as being with a loved one, taking the dog for a walk, sitting on the beach. Maybe this is something people without dementia should learn from people with dementia – the importance of appreciating and living for the moment, who knows what will happen tomorrow?

It is not only people with dementia who have stressed the need for this. Family carers have also documented the importance of appreciating the moment. (1)

The ability to recall long-term memories.

Most people know that dementia affects a person's ability to remember recent events, short-term memory. (This not the case for everyone with dementia –some people such as Graham mentioned earlier retain good recent memories). However many people with dementia will have an excellent ability to remember events from the past, their **long-term memory.**

One of our residents was a midwife. A member of staff, who was a midwife in the Philippines, showed a documentary about childbirth that had been on the TV. While Kath (the resident) watched the documentary she sobbed saying it brought back happy memories.

Quote from a Care home manager

Talking about the past, rather then the present can be easier for people. It can be tempting to ask people questions relating to the present as a way of stimulating conversation. Its something we all do with one another quite naturally e.g. asking if you have had a good day or discussing the terrible weather we are having. Yet for some people with dementia such questions rely too heavily on recent memories and so can cause great frustration for the person if they cannot remember. Instead use what you know about the person to ask questions about the past. Of course delving into a person's past can cause painful memories to resurface. If this is the case it is important to comfort the person as best you can.

It may seem strange that some people with dementia may not remember what happened recently but can still recall facts and information from years ago. To help understand why this is it is worth thinking of memories as a lane. As we grow we learn from our experiences and these are stored as memories to help us on our journey. Memories keep getting added and the lane keeps getting longer. At the end of the lane recent memories are stored, but the further we go back down the lane the older the memories are. In the brain recent memories are kept on the surface and old memories are stored deep in the brain.

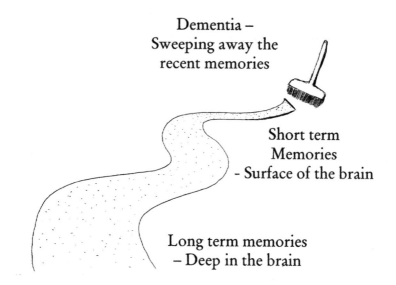

Dementia –
Sweeping away the
recent memories

Short term
Memories
- Surface of the brain

Long term memories
– Deep in the brain

Memory lane.

As dementia 'attacks' the surface of a person's brain it sweeps away some of the recent memories. The dementia has to 'brush away' more and more before it can get to the long term memories stored deep in the brain. Consequently the memories of a person's past are still there and so easier to recall.

The ability to connect with emotions.

People are not computers, we are SO MUCH more than machines storing facts and memories. Yet society seems to link our identity and self worth with what we can remember. We become so focused on the importance of remembering facts; we forget what makes us human, our **emotions.**

Recent research shown that the main part of the brain involved in emotions, the amygdala, stays relatively untouched by the advance of dementia. A consequence of this is that people with dementias emotional memory remains in tact. (A person's ability to recall feelings). Thus a person may forget recent events, because of their short term memory loss, but they will not forget how the event made them feel e.g., angry, happy, sad etc. This demonstrates why it is still important to involve a person with dementia with others and in activities. Even if they forget the conversation or the activity they will not forget how it made them feel – hopefully good!

People with dementia also seem to have an ability to pick up on people's thoughts and emotions by reading the non-verbal signals that people give.

I was so stressed. I was running late for work, I'd had an argument with my husband and I felt as if I was ready to explode. I walked through the doors of the ward and put on my 'happy face'. I said good morning to everyone as I walked to the nurse's station. A patient, a lady with dementia, who said very little, came over to me and took my hand. I protested that I didn't have time and I needed to get on. However her grip remained firm and slowly she walked me around the ward. At first I wanted to escape but I soon resigned myself to the fact she was not going to let go. I actually started to feel calmer. After a while she let go and carried on walking around the ward.

Quote from a Member of staff.

I have heard many descriptions from professionals and carers of their belief that many people with dementia can pick up on the feelings of another.

Despite the difficulties people with dementia face with communication, due to damage to the brain, they still have an amazing ability to find ways of communicating their needs and feelings. This is a great strength that is often not considered.

The ability to connect with others.

We are social animals – most of us need other people. This does not change by having dementia in fact it may mean that other people are needed now more than any other time in a person's life.

People with dementia still have the ability to relate and have relationships with others IF the right support is given to maintain these. Not having this in a person with dementia's life can lead to them becoming isolated.

The group I go to take you to the pub and a meal. I enjoy being with others who are in the same boat as me.

I have made new friends online.

I enjoy coming I get a lot out of these meetings.
Quotes from People with dementia

Professor Tom Kitwood, who developed the concept of person centred care for people with dementia, strongly argued that people with dementia are social beings. By this he meant that people with dementia have or have had a range of relationships with others. He conceptualised that it is these relationships that enable us to create our personhood. This is our identity, who we are. He went further to stress that if people with dementia continue to experience fulfilling relationships then their self-esteem and identity will be preserved.

The ability to stay active.

Many people with dementia remain physically active throughout their illness and the link between regular physical exercise and good health has been acknowledged for a long time.

I still like going for a walk when I can.

Quote from a Person with dementia.

Regular exercise helps a person with dementia to meet a number of their key needs including:

- Emotional Needs. Exercise can help in reducing feelings of stress and anxiety and can increase a person's self esteem.

- Social Needs. Group exercise such as Thai Chi or circle dance can help meet a person's social needs.

- Physical Health needs. Exercise helps prevent or reduce the risk of getting a number of other health problems.

Exercise does not need to be strenuous it can include things like:

- Household tasks such as dusting.
- Going for walks to the shops or places of interest
- Chair exercises.

Despite all of the benefits regular exercise brings people with dementia, its importance is often not considered.

For many people with dementia hobbies and activities are still an important part of keeping active. People may also enjoy social activities that involve others, such as music nights, sing-songs and dancing. These all promote relationships with others. Others may enjoy playing games, such as crossword puzzles, word games, quizzes, bingo or dominoes. However these games could cause some people with dementia to experience feelings of frustration. This is because these types of games rely on a person remembering a set of rules and the meaning of words or numbers. These games can be adapted to meet the individual needs of the person. However if it is felt that the games are causing frustration or distress for a person, it may be time to stop playing them.

Activities are only one way of occupying people with dementia. Many people with dementia may feel that they need to do something relating to their past role. For instance a person who was a homemaker may find tasks such as:

- making the bed,
- drying up,
- setting the table,
- dusting,
- watering pot plants

meets their needs, especially if they are asked to help. Furthermore people can feel busy and active without the help of others, as long as things are available for people to occupy themselves with. For instance you could have different tools for occupation around the home. This could include:

- Books and magazines.
- Different clothing such as hats, handbags and scarves.
- Dusters, a broom, a carpet sweeper.
- Tactile boards or trays.
- Bird feeders and a bird table in the garden.

The most important thing though is to provide an opportunity for the person with dementia to have fun, feel useful and maintain their strengths.

(1) McLay E (2006) Mom's OK, She Just Forgets: The Alzheimer's Journey from Denial to Acceptance. Prometheus Books.

This third chapter has considered some of the skills people with dementia may maintain. Next we attempt to explain what dementia is.

Chapter Four

What is Dementia?

Whether you have dementia or care for someone with dementia, learning about this condition can help considerably in understanding what is happening. However it is important to realise that there are no real experts in dementia, other then those who are living with it every day of their lives. As well as knowing the 'science' of dementia it is equally important, if not more important, to learn from people who are living with dementia. They will be able to give guidance and direction.

The first part of this chapter gives a definition of dementia followed by a description of what the anti-dementia drugs are.

Next the key causes of dementia are explored including Alzheimer's disease, vascular dementia, dementia with lewy bodies and the fronto-temporal dementias.

Then we discuss the process of diagnosis and the potential reasons why people develop dementia.

Finally this chapter details other forms of confusion and the difficulties this can cause.

What is dementia?

Soon after my Grandads' diagnosis he came to live with my parents and me. At the time I didn't really understand what was going on. I remember my parents talking about something called Alzheimer's but at that time in my life it meant very little to me. What I did know was the Grandad who used to help me build sandcastles on Bournemouth beach during happy family holidays now struggled to remember who I was.

It took me a long time before I understood the 'science' of dementia. I don't really know if this has helped me in my work with people who live with dementia and to truly understand who they are? Yet understanding what dementia is can be the first step in taking control. Consequently this chapter will focus on answering that very question - What is dementia?

I had a questionnaire from a charity and they kept interchanging the terms dementia and Alzheimer's and that really got my goat. Its like saying all vacuum cleaners are Dysons.

Quote from a Family carer

Dementia is not a disease in itself. Instead it is a term that doctors use to describe a group of symptoms. These symptoms can be caused by numerous illnesses that affect a person's brain. The main causes include

- Alzheimer's disease. (The commonest cause).
- Vascular dementia and
- Dementia with lewy bodies.

However not everyone will have the same symptoms and the intensity and duration of these symptoms will vary considerably from person to person. Symptoms can include a person experiencing gradual **changes** in their ability to:

- To remember recent events
- Find their way around in familiar places.
- Communicate or understand others.
- Think clearly.
- Carry out arithmetic.
- Undertake every day activities that the person once carried out with ease.
- Make judgements based on understanding risk and logic.

However this list of symptoms is not particular to dementia. These symptoms can be caused by other conditions, such as hypothyroidism (under active thyroid gland), brain tumours, vitamin deficiency and depression. The main difference between these conditions and dementia is that they can potentially be treated and so it is important that a person receives the correct diagnosis.

The Anti-dementia drugs.

There is currently no cure for the majority of the causes of dementia, including Alzheimer's disease. However there are a group of drugs called anti-dementia drugs or acetylcholinesterase inhibitors. They can help with some of the symptoms of Alzheimer's disease in some individuals.

Currently there are three anti-dementia drugs. These are:

- Donepezil (Aricept)
- Rivastigmine (Exelon)
- Galantamine (Reminyl)

Research has shown that people with Alzheimer's disease have a reduced level of a chemical called **Acetylcholine.** (This chemical is needed to help us learn, remember information and it is also involved in movement). Anti-dementia drugs work by stopping an enzyme, called Acetylcholinesterase, from breaking down Acetylcholine, increasing the amount of the memory chemical in a person's brain.

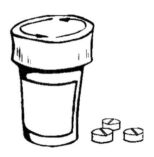

In the UK, due to a decision made by the National Institute of Clinical Excellence, these drugs are usually only used for people in the 'moderate stages' of Alzheimer's disease.

It's an outrage....my Dad has worked all his life. Now when he needs something back he can't get it.

Quote from a Family carer

I know not everyone benefits from these drugs. One of my residents had quite nasty side effects when she was taking it.

Quote from a Care Home Manager.

INFORMATION ABOUT DEMENTIA.

The numbers of people with dementia in the UK is currently estimated to be 700,000. This is expected to grow to over one million in 15 years time.

There are an estimated 17,000 younger people with dementia. i.e., people below the age of 65.

Old age is not a cause of dementia – however it is a risk factor. The older you are the more likely your are to develop dementia.

63% of people with dementia live in the community (1)

Worldwide, there is a new case of dementia every seven seconds. (2)

Everyone who has dementia will have a very different experience of their dementia.

Key causes of dementia:
Alzheimer's disease

The symptoms of Alzheimer's disease were first described by a German doctor, called Alois Alzheimer. He cared for a female patient, known as Auguste D, who was showing a number of symptoms, we now associate with Alzheimer's disease.

It absolutely exhausts me. Its like turning the tap on and watching it drain away.

All my thoughts are jumbled up.

I had to stop driving. I worried about my own safety and others.

Quotes from People with dementia.

After Auguste's death Dr Alzheimer's wanted to try and understand more about what had happened to her. He performed an examination of her brain, using a recently developed technique of tissue staining, to try and appreciate the possible causes of these symptoms. He found that numerous cells in Auguste's brain were seriously damaged. This damage was caused by deposits of bad protein known as **amyloid** and **tau.** (Even today it is not until a post mortem is performed of the brain that a diagnosis of Alzheimer's disease can be given for definite).

These deadly proteins gradually grow in number and wage a war against the person's brain cells and their connections. Tau protein attacks the cells from inside, causing tangles to form. This causes the cells to swell up like a balloon, until they explode and die. Amyloid protein causes plaques to form outside of the cell. These plaques then grow like ivy slowly suffocating the cell.

Working together, these plaques and tangles lead to certain areas of a person's brain being damaged. This damage firstly occurs in the memory part of the brain, hence the first symptom of short-term memory loss.

It is quite common to have a decline in our ability to remember, as we get older. This natural memory loss can be difficult to differentiate from the memory loss experienced early on in the dementia. However, later on in the dementia, increases in severity and the frequency of a person's memory difficulties becomes clearer. For instance forgetting the way home on a route that has been walked or driven hundreds of times before, or forgetting the name of a friend or family member, forgetting where you keep items in a kitchen you have used for years. **If you are worried about your memory it is important to go and see your doctor for advice.**

The plaques and tangles can spread to other parts of the brain resulting in the other symptoms of Alzheimer's, including personality changes, difficulties with walking and loss of mental abilities such as reading and writing.

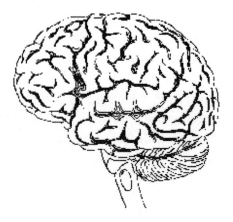

A picture showing a side view of the brain.

However each person's experience of Alzheimer's will be very different in its progression. For some the Alzheimer's will gradually progress over many years where others decline may be quicker.

It's a dodgy patch that he is going through but he seems to be levelling off.

They said to me that people with dementia can't sit with other people and they will be incontinent. I said to them that doesn't just happen with dementia.

Quotes from Family carers.

Vascular Dementia

There is a presumption that everyone has Alzheimer's but it's not the case.

Quotes from a Family carer.

Vascular dementia is a term used to describe a number of illnesses that affects the bodies' vascular system which results in a poor blood supply to the brain. Our brain needs this supply of blood to provide it with oxygen and nutrients. The vascular system does this by sending blood to the brain via a network of arteries.

For the oxygenated blood to get to the brain an unobstructed path is needed with a healthy heart to pump it there. Consequently heart disease, high blood pressure or blockages to the arteries can affect the blood supply and so cause cells in the brain to starve to death leading to vascular dementia, as illustrated in the next diagram.

See below.

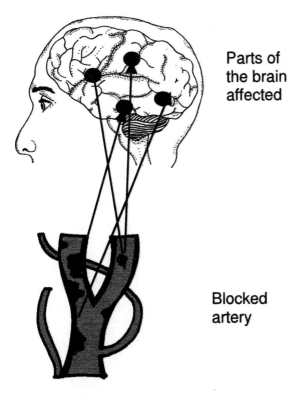

Parts of the brain affected

Blocked artery

The commonest cause of vascular dementia is a stroke. A stroke happens when a blockage in an artery stops the blood getting to the brain or when the artery itself becomes damaged. This causes the brain cells to die or become damaged and causes the symptoms of dementia.

After the stroke he became very low. He wouldn't even talk to his best friend who he had known for years.

It was heart breaking to see what was happening to him.

He is always lost in the house, he can't put a plug in a socket, he's lost all his skills. The only control he's got at the moment is whether he gets a hair cut and what he eats.

He's changed a lot over the past 6-8 weeks. He's really down because Tom knows he has changed but he can't do anything about it. He's not the same person he was.

Quotes from Family Carers

The symptoms of vascular dementia often depend on which area of the brain has been affected and how badly damaged this area is.

In the early stages of vascular dementia a person may not experience the same memory difficulties as in Alzheimer's disease and so have a greater awareness of the difficulties they are experiencing. Such difficulties can include:

- Problems with walking.
- Problems with communication such as slurred speech.
- Becoming withdrawn, either because of communication problems or a loss of confidence.
- Symptoms that are linked to strokes such as paralysis.

It is potentially possible to help a person with vascular dementia by encouraging them to:

- Stop smoking
- Take regular exercise.
- Follow a healthy diet.

A person with vascular dementia should also have their blood pressure regularly checked by their GP. Their GP may also prescribe the person medication, such as Non-steroidal anti-inflammatory agents (NSAIDs), hypotensives or statins, to try and reduce the risk of further strokes occurring.

Dementia with Lewy Bodies

A colleague of Alois Alzheimer's, Dr Friedrich Heinrich Lewy, first described an abnormal build up of protein, known as lewy bodies, which destroys brain cells and leads to a form of dementia called Dementia with Lewy bodies.

People with dementia with lewy bodies can have similar symptoms to both Alzheimer's disease (memory problems) and Parkinson's disease (problems with movement and balance which can result in the person having a number of falls). Dementia with lewy bodies also has other symptoms including hallucinations.

I've had quite a running battle with a couple of things. I see a group of line dancers who haunt me.

The strangest things have scared me. I was in bed in the middle of the night and we've got a portable television in the bedroom.

Between me and it (the television) we had an argument. I know it sounds ridiculous and people will say I am crazy. It scared the life out of me.

It's hard when I see things that are disturbing.

Quotes from people with dementia with lewy bodies.

It has also been suggested that in this type of dementia a person can experience a fluctuation of abilities throughout the day.

In Parkinson's disease, lewy bodies are usually found in the brain stem where they attack a chemical called dopamine. This causes symptoms of Parkinson's disease such as rigidity, stiffness and tremors. However Dr Lewy found that in some cases these lewy bodies spread to other parts of the brain, which caused the symptoms of dementia. Hence the name dementia with lewy bodies. (Parkinson's disease is not a type of dementia however some people with Parkinson's will go on to develop dementia, which is similar to Dementia with Lewy bodies).

The Fronto-temporal dementias.

Fronto-temporal dementia relates to a number of different dementias the most common being Picks disease.

My dad has Picks. He has changed from a kind, caring father to someone I don't even recognise.

Quote from a Family carer

Picks disease was identified by a doctor, called Arnold Pick. He discovered that in the brains of people with this type of dementia that their cells were unusual in shape and swollen. He called these cells Pick cells. Also Dr Pick identified a build up of protein, which he called Pick bodies. As in the plaques and tangles, seen in Alzheimer's disease, these Pick bodies and Pick cells work together to cause the death of a person's cells located in the front part of the brain.

Initially in Pick's disease a person's personality and behaviour will be affected before their short-term memory. This is different to Alzheimer's disease where short-term memory problems is the first symptom.

Diagnosis

Diagnosis of dementia by clinicians is not an easy process. Multiple tests can be undertaken although no one test can give a definite answer. Doctors may undertake memory tests such as the Mini Mental State Examination (MMSE). This involves asking the person numerous questions that tests their memory, language and mathematical ability.

The Psychiatrist doing the MMSE asked the person to write down the first thing that came into their head. The person wrote, "Shut up man".

Quote from a Care home manager.

A person may have brain scans and blood tests or urine tests to rule out other conditions that could be causing the symptoms shown. Often health and social care professionals will use jargon and acronyms (see chart below) to describe what is happening. So don't feel embarrassed about asking questions if you don't understand what is being said. One carer I worked with always took a tape recorder with her when she went to the doctors with her husband. If there was anything that she did not understand or forgot she could listen to the recording again. Other carers have suggested writing down the questions you want to ask before visiting the doctors.

Acronym	What it stands for.
CPN	Community Psychiatric Nurse or Community Mental Health Nurses have had extra training to work in the field of mental health and work in the community.
CMHT	Community Mental Health Team. There are a number of community mental health teams (CMHT) for older people around the country. These are group of different professionals including psychiatrists; clinical psychologists and community mental health nurses that provide psychological support for people with severe mental illness. Although some CMHT's provide support for people with dementia, this is not the case for all teams. In certain areas of the country a person with dementia may be referred to a memory clinic. This is also a team of specialists however, rather then focusing on a wide range of mental illnesses they specialise in dementia and other causes of severe memory loss.
RMN	Registered Mental Nurse. They will care for a person

	with dementia if they are is admitted to a mental health hospital or ward.
OT	Occupational therapists advise on ways of maintaining independence for as long as possible, by adaptations of the existing environment and through additional equipment that is available.
PCT.	Primary Care Trusts are NHS organisations that employ staff who are based in or visit people in the local community such as, General Practitioners and Practice Nurses. (A nurse that works mainly in a doctor's surgery). Trusts can go on to 'purchase' secondary care for people who need further support. For example the GP may decide that a person with dementia needs to go into hospital to see a specialist.
MMSE	Mini Mental State Examination. A test used to assess a person's ability to recall information.
CQC	Care Quality Commission. The CQC regulate, inspect and review all adult health and social care services in the public, private and voluntary sectors in England.
Admiral Nurses.	These individuals specialise in working with people with dementia and their carers. They can provide information, practical advice and help other professionals to deliver positive care. Admiral Nurses Direct is an advice and support line and can be called on 0845 257 9406 or emailed on direct@dementiauk.org

What causes dementia?

For the majority of the forms of dementias we still do not know the cause, although there have been numerous suggestions. It is suspected that dementia may be caused by a combination of factors, such as genetics and social factors. One of the key factors to be aware of is that having dementia is not the person's fault. There is nothing that the person has done that has caused them to have dementia.

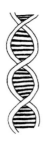

DNA Structure

It is thought that genetics may play a strong part in some cases. Research has looked at a number of chromosome's including numbers 21, 19, 14, and 10. For instance Familial Alzheimer's disease (FAD) is a type of Alzheimer's disease where the cause seems to be genetic. Yet this type of Alzheimer's disease only accounts for about 5 – 10% of total cases.

There are many cases where no one else in the family has had dementia. This means that there must be other reasons why people develop dementia other than just genetics.

Suggestions for other possible causes cover a wide spectrum including pollution, problems with the immune system and head injuries however the research is still inconclusive.

What we do know is that dementia is not caused by old age, as it was once thought. We know this because anyone of any age can have dementia. There are about 17,000 below the age of 65 with dementia in the UK. There have been cases of children having dementia caused by conditions such as Neimans' Pick Disease type C. (A very rare genetic disease) However age is a risk factor, the older you are the more likely you are to have dementia. For instance one person in twenty aged over 65 will have dementia however this increases quite dramatically to one in three people over the age of 90.

Other forms of confusion.

Certain conditions can make it even harder for people with dementia to remember things and can make them even more confused. Causes of increased confusion can include:

- Medication or drugs, including alcohol.
- Infections such as urine or chest infections.
- Poor diet.
- Constipation.
- Shock.
- Dehydration.
- Head injuries.

These causes of confusion are known as *acute* confusion. This means that, with help, this confusion should only be short term. It is important that acute confusion is dealt with to make sure that the person with dementia does not have to experience increased confusion for any longer than is necessary.

(1)The National Audit Office (2007) Improving services and support for people with dementia

(2)Ferri et al (2005) Global prevalence of dementia: a Delphi consensus study. The Lancet 366, 2112-2117

The next chapter will go on to discuss how people with dementia use their behaviour as a form of communication to express a need.

****

Chapter Five

Behaviour: a Form of Communication.

Having dementia can often influence a person's behaviour. This can be one of the hardest challenges faced by people living with dementia. Often families describe caring for someone who shows difficult behaviour as a major challenge and this can put a great deal of strain on the relationship.

Firstly this chapter illustrates that behaviour is a trait of humanity and not just a symptom of dementia, as suggested by the medical model.

Secondly we look at the different reasons that may be causing a person's behaviour.

Then we examine different types of behaviour, in closer detail. Including aggression, repetitiveness and wandering.

Finally the importance of looking for triggers is reflected upon.

Behaviours are a human trait.

The medical model has presumed that the behaviour shown by people with dementia is a symptom of dementia and thus is an inevitable part of their illness. The new culture of care has suggested that, as with all of us, people with dementia will use their behaviour as a form of communication. (It may be the only language they have left to tell others about a need).

We all express behaviours, who hasn't paced around because they are nervous or angry, who hasn't shouted at someone because they were upset or scared?

The key difference between people without dementia and those with dementia is that their behaviour cannot be controlled in the same way. The judgement of people with dementia, their self-control and ability to follow social rules has been affected due to damage to the brain. This does not prevent the behaviour being any less difficult or worrying, but it does show that this behaviour is not deliberate, although it may feel like it at times.

Reasons for behaviour.

There can numerous reasons for a person's behaviour. This could be linked to:

Their past. All of us are affected by our past, it gives us an insight into how to act in certain situations. Often a person with dementia will be significantly influenced by the role they played in their life, including their parental and occupational roles. Some people's behaviour may be related to a previous hobby or skill.

Pain & discomfort. When we need help because we feel unwell all we have to do is ask. However for people with dementia, because of problems with speech, they may have to rely heavily on their behaviour to communicate.

Medication. The side effects of a person's medication could be causing the behaviour.

Others. Other people will influence a person's behaviour especially if they are asked to do something they can not do or are made to feel foolish or inadequate.

It was always a different carer who would come. I didn't feel that I could challenge the carers if I thought they were misunderstanding my husband.

Quote from a Family carer.

I've been encouraged to go to a group and there are about a dozen people who are at a different level to me. They're going through hard times. I don't enjoy it because of this. I have said to my wife that I am not going anymore but she told me that we had to wait a long time before I could get into this group.

Quote from a Person with dementia.

A person's surroundings. A person's environment will influence their behaviour. For example loud noise could be a source of distress.

Changes in the brain.

Another possible reason behind a person's behaviour is due to the changes that have occurred in the brain. Damage to a person's brain prevents it from working as it should, which can lead to a number of behaviours occurring.

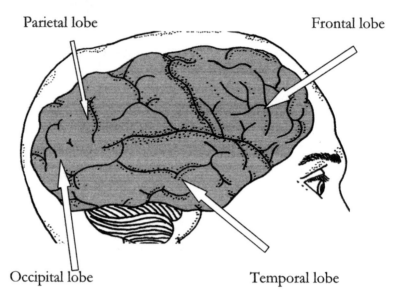

Parietal lobe

Frontal lobe

Occipital lobe

Temporal lobe

Diagram showing the four main parts of the brain.

The Frontal Lobe.

The front part of the brain is called the Frontal lobe. If this part of the brain becomes damaged, because of the dementia, it may affect a person's ability to follow and understand social rules and consequently their ability to make judgments about how to 'act' in certain situations.

Consequently a person's sexual behaviour may become more explicit or a person's understanding of social eating may alter. They may undress in front of others, without realising that it is 'socially inappropriate' to do so in this situation.

If a person undresses in a socially inappropriate setting, the first instinct may be to tell the person off or to tell them to stop it or highlight to the person that they have behaved in this way. However this may not be helpful. This is because damage to their short-term memory will reduce the person's ability to learn new information. A person may forget what has been said and only remember the feelings they are left with, an emotional memory.

Yet it is worth considering why the person has behaved in this way. Is it because the person:

- Is too hot or cold?
- Is uncomfortable in the clothes they are wearing?
- Needs to use the toilet?
- Does not realise that there are others in the room?

Damage to the frontal lobe can cause the person to have problems with:

- Making decisions, such as what to wear, what time to catch a bus, what to do in an emergency etc.
- Planning how to get somewhere, how to cook a meal or what to do to keep busy.
- Solving problems such as deciding how to overcome obstacles, who to call if in trouble.

The Temporal Lobe

Another part of the brain that can be affected in dementia is the temporal lobe. The temporal lobe contains a part of the brain known as the hippocampus. This small area of the brain is involved both in memory and spatial navigation. (Being able to get us around without becoming lost).

In Alzheimer's disease it is the hippocampus that is affected first which explains the early symptoms of disorientation and memory loss. You might see a person with dementia showing a number of behaviours associated with short- term memory problems, such as repeating themselves or walking around and around.

The Parietal Lobe

This part of the brain is mainly involved with making sense of sensory information, such as sound, touch and taste. The parietal lobe also helps us to use and understand language. If this part of the brain becomes damaged, a person can have major problems with language. This can cause great frustration for people with dementia. Damage to this area may explain why some people with dementia repeat themselves – because they cannot make sense of the answers they are given.

The Occipital Lobe.

The occipital lobe helps us to make sense of what we see around us. Damage to this part of the brain will influence how a person sees the world. For instance a person might:

- Misinterpret a floral pattern in a carpet as an animal or a face.
- On a black and white floor the person may see the black squares as holes and so refuse to walk on the floor.

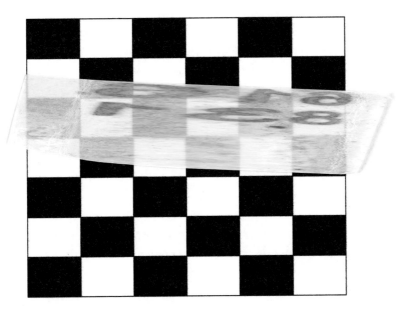

- Not see the toilet because the white toilet seat, the white toilet and the white floor all blend into one.

- Take a large step over a join in the flooring because they think it is a step.

If you have all the halls the same colour the person's got no chance. Its simple, colour code the corridors to help people orientate themselves.

Quote from a Family carer.

Consequently how a person's brain *'sees'* the surroundings can cause a person's behaviour. However, it may be possible to stop some of these behaviors by adapting a person's environment, just as you would for other disabilities. For instance by:

- Replacing patterned curtains, floor coverings, soft furnishings etc with plain ones.
- Replacing white toilet seats with black toilet seats.
- Using clear signs / pictures on doors.
- Having distinct differences between the walls and floors through use of colours and textures.
- Providing circular paths around the garden or in the home to stop the person being faced with constant dead ends.

The key thing is that a person with dementia's environment can be changed to support them and suit their needs.

A person with dementia may also have problems with the environment if they are relying heavily on their long-term memory. For instance a person may not recognise a modern push down flush on a toilet because they are used to a chain flush.

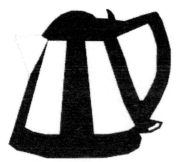

The person may put an electric kettle on the hob because that's the way they used to be. In cases like this it might be an idea to buy a kettle that can be used in this way rather then leaving the electric kettle out.

Different types of behaviour:
Aggression

He is deemed as dangerous now but he's not. I'm still his little girl. When he sees me he doesn't know my name but he still calls me his little sausage.

Quote from a Family carer.

Probably the behaviour carers find most difficult to handle is aggression; this is often because the consequences of an aggressive act can have a long lasting affect on a carer both physically and emotionally. These affects can be magnified if the person with dementia has never showed aggression before the illness.

Aggression can also affect the person with dementia. If a person remembers being aggressive they may struggle to understand why they have acted this way, especially if it is a change in their personality. Even if a person can't remember they may be only too aware of the fall out after the incident.

Dealing with aggressive behaviour is not easy and no one can say for certain what is the best way of managing aggression; however here are some factors to consider.

- Raising your voice, shouting at the person or arguing with the person may only make the matter worse.

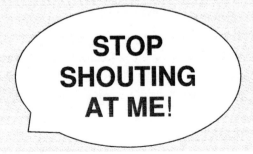

- Telling a person to 'calm down' will most likely cause the person to do the opposite.

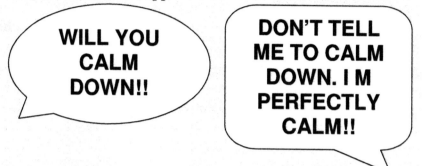

- Give the person lots of space. The person probably won't appreciate being touched until the feelings of anger have gone.

- Tell the person that you are not going to harm them. (they might be being aggressive because they believe you are going to harm them).

- Listen to what the person is saying.

- Try to divert their attention onto something else.

- Try and keep yourself calm. This will be difficult because your heart will probably be pounding because of the emotions you are feeling, however this is vital if the person with dementia is to calm down also.

- Punishing or scolding a person for being aggressive may not be helpful because they will forget both the incident of aggression and the resulting punishment. However they may not forget the *feelings* the punishment created in them, possibly anger. This anger then may build through out the day until it is again expressed through aggression.

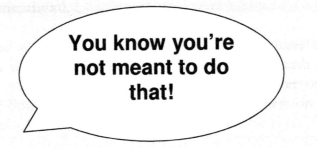

Anger can be a good thing, it is what makes us stand up for ourselves. However when anger turns into violence this is not good. For some people with dementia they may not have chance to express their anger and consequently it builds into violence, a bit like steam in a kettle. If it does not have opportunity to be released in small controlled amounts then it will boil over.

A person with dementia can be helped to release their anger in a controlled way, through things such as exercise. This will not help everyone but may be useful for some.

Supporting someone with dementia can be incredibly hard work, especially if you are not getting any or very little support yourself. As a family member it is ok to be honest with the person with dementia and others and tell them that you are feeling angry or annoyed. However if you feel that your anger is building into violence then you need to find strategies to help with this.

As a family member you don't have to deal with this on your own. If you are worried tell your doctor or contact your local branch of the Alzheimer's society for advice.

The house feels so empty, even though he's still living with me.

Quote from a Family carer.

Repetitiveness

Repetitiveness refers to when a person with dementia repeats a word, phrase or action.

She went through a stage of saying the same thing over and over again. That drained me more than the physical violence.

Quote from a Family carer.

A person with dementia may have genuinely forgotten either asking the question or the answer they received, and if greeted with an angry response, may see this as an unreasonable reaction to a question. People try and cope with this in different ways. Some people have a written answer for the person with dementia to read, some people try diverting the person's attention on to something else and others have considered there is meaning behind the words repeated (see chapter 6).

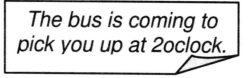

Wandering.

Carers often find a person's wandering particularly distressing especially if the person with dementia wanders away from home at night.

You meet people, you have things to see.

I suddenly realised I didn't know where the hell I was. I realised I had to do something. I thought if I head for the main road I am bound to get somewhere which I did. It took a long time to get home.

Quotes from people with dementia.

He has always walked...but this does not stop me from worrying what will happen to him when he is out there.

They suggested a tracker device that we could use. So we have acquired one and I'm still getting to grips with it. I text the tracker device and it sends me back the coordinates of where he is on a map.

When he did get lost and I had to call the police and I was so impressed the way there was no judgement. After three hours I called them and explained that he had dementia and he had been gone be for three hours. Within about twenty minutes I got a call from the local police station who then came out to the house.

Mike can't get himself dressed anymore and he's up and down during the night. He gets up to all sorts of things...it doesn't bear thinking about.

I can't take her far. She gets too tired and her mobility's not to good, she wanders about all over the place.

Quotes from Family carers

Although to the observer wandering may seem aimless there is often a reason behind the person's walking. This could include:

- Boredom. We all need to keep physically active and stimulated otherwise we become bored. If you think this is the reason behind the person's walking try and find something to prevent boredom. Consider activities that the person used to enjoy. These may be work related activities.

I've worked with children all of my life but now I don't see any.

Quote from a Person with dementia.

- Pain. People may be walking to try and relieve pain or physical discomfort. It is worth watching a person's body language to see if they look in discomfort. Ask the person if they are in pain. If this is the case contact the person's doctor for advice.

- Searching. The person may have forgotten when they last saw a person or where they put an item so they may be walking around to try and find something or someone.

I'm up most of the day looking for this, looking for that.
Quote from a Person with dementia.

- New environment. When a person with dementia comes to a new environment they may be walking around to try and understand where they are. In the person's own environment it is worth considering the use of signs on doors, particularly for the toilet. Use both words and pictures on the signs as illustrated here.

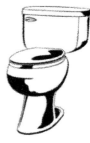

- Disorientation between night and day. A person may be getting up in the night because they believe it is daytime. Consider buying a large traditional clock or a digital clock with AM and PM on them.

I think they worry about me because they think I am going to get lost. I am not as useless as they think.
Quote from a Person with dementia.

Accepting a person's mistakes.

It hit me like a train. I had spent so much time battling with him, pointing out when he got it wrong. I realised this was the source of our arguments. Yes it annoyed the hell out of me that he couldn't put his socks away in the right place or that he used his fingers more often then his knife and fork. It became easier when I learnt to bite my tongue, which trust me was not always easy!
Quote from a Family carer

A family member talked to me about the importance of accepting that nobody gets *'it'* perfect 100% of the time. She explained that a great source of frustration for her early on in her husband's dementia was his inability to put things away in the correct area, for instance socks in the wrong draw, milk in the freezer and so on.

Highlighting to him his mistake was often a cause of many arguments and so her husband was becoming verbally aggressive.

Working with a support group, run by the local Alzheimer's society, enabled her to understand why her husband was doing this (not to annoy her as she originally thought) and to realise that pointing out his mistakes did not help. Instead she learnt that the socks could always be moved later on or a pint of milk could be salvaged, which was much easier then trying to salvage her husbands dented pride.

Looking for Triggers.

When considering the reasons behind a person's behaviour it is worth thinking about what triggered or caused the behaviour. A trigger is something used to describe anything that causes a person's behaviour. This could include:

- Being in a noisy room.
- Another individual has shouted at the person
- The person with dementia does not know where they are.
- The person is asked to do something they can't do.

Writing a diary of the behaviours shown may allow a pattern to emerge of when each behaviour occurs.

In the last chapter the importance of communication is looked at.

****

Chapter Six

Keep listening!

Some people with dementia may have problems with their speech during their journey of dementia. For many people without dementia it can be difficult to interact with a person who loses their speech. Consequently this final chapter looks at the importance of good communication and its role in helping maintain the relationship between those without dementia and a person with.

The first part of this chapter looks at the need to listen and the different techniques that can be used to demonstrate listening.

Then the importance of looking for meaning behind the words and sounds is explored.

The chapter finishes by considering how communication can be used to help a person make decisions.

The importance of being listened to.

It's as if when you got this label that you give people permission to ignore you.

I don't think she realised how much people with dementia in the group could talk – we will say what we want to say and I think it frightened her.

People's sympathy runs out and they can't maintain that level of engagement.

You talking to me is great. That's what I need right now.

Quotes from People with dementia.

As the above quotes suggest people with dementia are not listened to. The issue is if people are not listened to then their feelings of value and self worth will be affected. However by something as simple as listening to a person with dementia we can give a person's self esteem a massive boost.

SHOWING the person that you are listening to them is important. Even if you can't understand what the person is saying you can still show the person that you are listening and so acknowledge the person's worth.

Experts in reading non-verbal communication.

Communication allows people to exchange thoughts, ideas and information by using different methods. There are verbal forms of communication and nonverbal methods. Verbal communication usually refers to the sending or receiving of words, for example through speech or sign language. Non verbal communication refers to when we send or receive wordless messages. This can be done through body language, facial expressions and so on.

At what point does anybody actually listen to what I want?
Quote from a Person with dementia.

Because of the difficulties a person with dementia may face with words, they may rely heavily on non-verbal forms of communication. Although they may lose the meaning of words the feelings behind them will still be understood by reading what you are communicating non verbally. Therefore people with dementia can become EXPERTS in reading non-verbal communication. Consequently, when you are with a person with dementia, you need to be very aware of the signals you are sending to the person. Think about your tone of voice, your facial expressions and your body language. Consider if you are showing that you are listening to a person through your non-verbal communication. This can be done through:

- Eye contact – I believe there is truth in the old saying 'eyes are the window of the soul". People with dementia may try and figure out what is being said by looking at your eyes. Using eye contact shows to the person that you are paying attention and you have shown you are interested.

- Posture – arms folded indicates you are shutting the other person out.

- Facial expressions – your face needs to show that you're listening. Yawning kind of gives it away that you're not interested!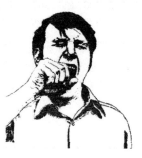

- Positioning – Sit in a position where the person can easily see you, don't stand over the person or talk over the person.
- Meaningful touch – indicates care and understanding, however this does have to be **meaningful** to the individual. Some people will respond well to touch where as others may find it intrusive.

- Proximity – how physically close are you to the person? Are you too close so that they feel uncomfortable?

- Reflective listening – responding to, and describing in different words, your understanding of what the person with dementia has said.

- Tone of voice. Even if the person with dementia does not understand what you are saying they will get an impression of what you are saying by listening to your voice. Tone, pitch, speed and volume all gives indicators to the person of what you are saying and how you are feeling. For example the words 'don't worry about it' can be said with anger or with an understanding tone.

- Mirroring. This involves observing the person's body language and reflecting this in your own body language. For example if a person was to smile you could smile also. However be careful that mirroring does not turn into copying everything the person does.

- Silence. Don't feel awkward if there are moments of silence. We all need these periods of quiet to reflect upon what has been said or is about to be said.

- Using short sentences. If your sentences are too long then the person with dementia may lose track of what you are saying.

- Reducing questions that test short-term memory. Because a person with dementia is likely to have problems recalling recent memories asking questions such as, *'what have you had for lunch'?* or *'where have you been today'?* may cause the person frustration and embarrassment because they don't know the answer.

- Giving people time to respond. For some people with dementia it may take them longer to respond to what is being asked. It can be tempting to ask a person another question if we don't get an immediate response from an initial question but give the person opportunity to respond.

It's interesting to see how she will bring a topic that she is familiar with into what you're talking about because that's what she's comfortable with.
My mum in the conversation looks for links, like we all do, but she will make really bizarre links.

He likes to talk about experiences from the war mainly.

Quotes from Family members.

It is also useful to consider factors that may make it easier for the person with dementia to communicate with others. For instance be aware of noise levels. (It's quite hard to talk to somebody in a very noisy setting).

Meaning behind the words.

Some people with dementia may ask for deceased parents or spouses. Others may talk about picking their adult 'children' up from school or say they need to go to work even though they are retired. There are a number of possible approaches when responding to such questions.

- *Tell the truth.*

- *Going along with.*

- *Distraction.*

- *Looking for meaning.*

Tell the truth.

For some people with dementia it may be appropriate to tell them the real situation e.g. That there children have grown up or their mother/ father has passed away. However you should tell this information in a sensitive way – if possible.

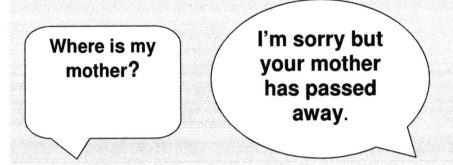

Yet the difficulty comes when a person is regularly confronted with the reality. If a person is frequently asking the same question and is being told the truth through out the day then this may cause the person great distress.

The damage to a person's memory means they may forget information including the loss of the parent or that they are retired. When a person is told the reality they experience the loss as if it was for the first time and so feel the pain that goes with the realisation of the truth.

Going along with it.

Another approach is going along with the person's reality. For instance if a person asks when her mother is coming you could say *"your mother is coming later today"*. This may work for some people with dementia but for others they may realise that you are not telling the truth.

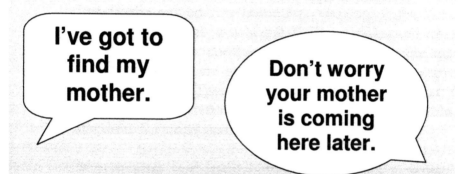

In a situation like this it is important that everyone has the same response to the person's answers. If one person tells them that their mother is dead and another states that she is coming along later this will only lead to more confusion and distress.

Distraction.

In this case you could try different things to distract the person, e.g. asking the person if they would like a drink or discuss subjects relating to the person who they are asking for.

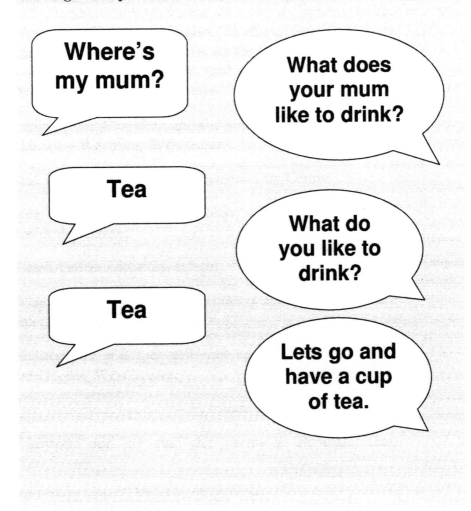

Where's my mum?

What does your mum like to drink?

Tea

What do you like to drink?

Tea

Lets go and have a cup of tea.

Looking for meaning

Another possibility is that when a person is talking about something from their past it may in fact relate to their current emotions. Think about the words the person is using, for instance are they asking for their mother because they need someone to undertake the same role that their mother did, making them feel secure, loved and comforted. (For many of us there is a significant person we turn to in times of trouble whether it is our children, our parents, friends or partners).

Another example is when a person believes that they are still working when in reality they have retired. By saying that they are going to work they could be trying to tell others that they need to experience how work used to make them feel e.g. involved, engaged and useful.

Bill was a retired farmer living in our care home. Since his childhood he had lived and worked on a farm and he believed that he was still there. My staff initially encouraged Bill to take it easy and enjoy his retirement but this contradicted his belief that he had to collect his chicken's eggs. The difference in realities between Bill and the staff soon led to conflict. Consequently we decided to buy some chickens. Bill collected the eggs everyday, which kept him happy and busy.
Quote from a Care home manager

If you believe that the person is discussing current feelings consider how you could help the person to meet these emotions. Just listening to the person, rather then disagreeing or agreeing with them can often help.

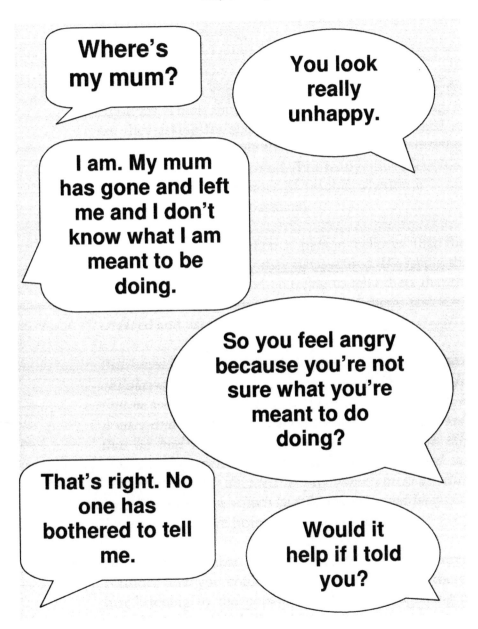

This approach is much more then verbal language. Listen to the person's tone of voice; does it give you a clue about how the person is feeling? Observe a person's body language and facial expression, will this help you see the emotions behind the person's words?

Use the communication skills, discussed earlier, to show that you are listening to the person.

Meaningful sounds.

I could tell how hard he was trying to tell me from the look on his face.

Quote from a Family member

There may be a point when a person with dementia can only express a few words or sounds. It is vital to recognise that despite the belief of the medical model, that these sounds are nothing more than a jumble of nonsense, that there is meaning to them.

If people believe that these words and sounds are meaningless then others may avoid talking to that person. If this happens then a person will not have the opportunity to express their communication and so may lose this ability altogether.

So even if what the person says seems to make little sense it is still essential to try and involve the person in conversation and show that you are listening. At least they still have the ability to use sound.

Using communication to help with decision-making.

People with dementia often have decisions made for them, even if they can make these decisions themselves. It is believed that the person is not able to make valued choices because of their illness.

There will be certain decisions that you and others may need to make. Nevertheless it is still important to allow the person to have as much control over their life as possible. Otherwise the person will lose their self-respect and feelings of worth.

Therefore you will need to use your communication skills effectively to enable people to take an active role in their care. For example, frustration can be caused by asking a question such as, *"What would you like to wear today"*? This is because the person has to try and remember what clothes they own and which clothes are appropriate for the day?

If this does cause frustration, then you could:

- Choose two items of clothing for the person, e.g. two dresses.

- Show them to the person and

- Ask, *"Would you like to wear this dress or this dress"*?

The person could be helped further by:

- Labelling drawers where items are kept.

- Laying the clothes out in the order the person will put them on.

- Handing clothes to the person as each item is required.

- Maintaining the person's dignity at each stage of dressing.

This final chapter has explored the importance of maintaining meaningful communication.

****

Final words

Whether you have dementia yourself or are supporting a person with dementia I hope this book has brought you some ideas about how to live well with dementia. You may have found from reading the book that some parts have particularly resonated with your own experience where as others have not. Hopefully those pieces that were useful will keep you thinking about your own situation long after you have put the book down?

You may be reading this book during some of your darkest days during the journey of dementia, when you feel depressed or believe there is no future. But trust me there will be a time when you realise that you and the people around you have made steps forward on the journey.

In my journey I have found a number of books very useful and you may find them helpful too. These include:

- Carol Simpson's book called, *"At the heart of Alzheimer's"*. Published by Manor Healthcare Corp.

- Joanne Koenig Coste's book called, *"Learning to Speak Alzheimer's – the new approach to living positively with Alzheimer's disease"*. Published by Vermilion – London.

- John Zeisel's book called, *"I'm still here- a breakthrough approach to understanding someone living with Alzheimer's"*. Published by Piatkus.

The battle ahead.

For all of us, with or without dementia, we face many key battles ahead in making sure that everyone lives WELL with dementia, whether you are a person with dementia or a carer or a family member. Some of those will be very personal, others on a national level.

Nationally we face the challenge of making sure that the National dementia strategy is not ignored by our politicians or individuals working in health and social care and is that it remains a high priority.

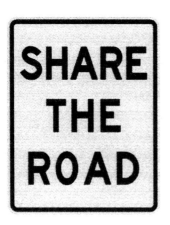

Despite the future battles we face there have been major steps forward. To reiterate what was written in chapter two, many people's perception about dementia has started to change for the better. More services are now focusing on the person and their needs rather then the restricted ideas of the past. A more 'balanced view' of dementia is being used within the media. More people living with dementia are openly talking about their experiences.

All of this can only help in changing societies view about dementia. People living with dementia have shown us that having dementia can remind us of what really matters in life – each other.

David

Useful Contacts

Alzheimer's Society,
Devon House, 58 St Katharine's Way. London E1W 1JX
020 7423 3500
Email enquiries@alzheimers.org.uk   www.alzheimers.org.uk/

Alzheimer Scotland,
22 Drumsheugh Gardens,
Edinburgh. EH3 7RN
Phone: 0131 243 1453.
E-mail: alzheimer@alzscot.org.   www.alzscot.org.uk

The Alzheimer's Research Trust.
The Stables, Station Road, Great Shelford,
Cambridge. CB22 5LR
Phone: 01223 843899
enquiries@alzheimers-research.org.uk
www.alzheimers-research.org.uk

The Picks Disease Support Group
8 Brooksby Close, Oadby,
Leicester. LE2 5AB
Phone: 0116 271 1414
info@pdsg.org.uk   www.pdsg.org.uk

CJD Support Network.
PO Box 346, Market Drayton,
Shropshire TF9 4WN
Phone: 01630 673 993

Lewy Body Society
info@lewybody.org.   www.lewybody.org

The Clive project
PO Box 315, Witney,
Oxfordshire. OX28 1ZN
Phone: 01993 776295
mail@thecliveproject.org.uk

Dementia UK
6 Camden High Street
London
NW1 0JH
Tel: 020 7874 7210
Fax: 020 7874 7219
E-mail: info@dementiauk.org

Age UK
Astral House
1268 London Road, London SW16 4ER
Phone: **020 8765 7200**
Email: contact@ageuk.org.uk

Index

Emerald Publishing
www.emeraldpublishing.co.uk

106 Ladysmith Road
Brighton BN2 4EG

Other titles in the Emerald Series:

Law
Guide to Bankruptcy
Conducting Your Own Court case
Guide to Consumer law
Creating a Will
Guide to Family Law
Guide to Employment Law
Guide to European Union Law
Guide to Health and Safety Law
Guide to Criminal Law
Guide to Landlord and Tenant Law
Guide to the English Legal System
Guide to Housing Law
Guide to Marriage and Divorce
Guide to The Civil Partnerships Act
Guide to The Law of Contract
The Path to Justice
You and Your Legal Rights

Health
Guide to Combating Child Obesity
Asthma Begins at Home

Natures Health Secret's series:

Remedies from the Sea
Reversing osteoarthritis
Natures Aspirin
Detox naturally

Music
How to Survive and Succeed in the Music Industry

General
A Practical Guide to Obtaining probate
A Practical Guide to Residential Conveyancing
Writing The Perfect CV
Keeping Books and Accounts-A Small Business Guide
Business Start Up-A Guide for New Business
Finding Asperger Syndrome in the Family-A Book of Answers

For details of the above titles published by Emerald go to:

www.emeraldpublishing.co.uk

Other Titles in the Emerald Explaining Series

EXPLAINING
AUTISM SPECTRUM DISORDER
Clare Lawrence

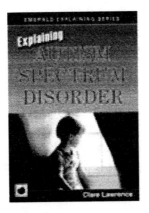

What is Autism Spectrum Disorder? With Autism and Asperger syndrome now reckoned to affect one in a hundred of our population, this is a question that more and more people are needing to ask.

'Explaining Autism Spectrum Disorder' is the first book in a new series, the 'Explaining' series and provides a clear and concise introduction to this fascinating and perplexing subject. Written in accessible, non-specialist language it provides an ideal introduction for parents, carers, teachers and employers – for anyone coming across this intriguing condition – on ways to understand what is the Autistic Spectrum.

The book covers:
- The 'Triad of Impairment'
- Getting a diagnosis
- Sensory issues
- Special interests
- Anxiety, depression and anger
- Ways to provide support
- Encouraging friendships
- Living with - and celebrating - the condition

The book includes a comprehensive section on managing school, and gives pointers for parents and carers, and for adults with autism themselves, on pathways to help and support.

The Author: Clare Lawrence is a teacher and a mother of two children, one of whom has autism. She is a graduate of Oxford, York, Northumbria, Sheffield Hallam and Birmingham universities, has a University Certificate in Autism Spectrum Disorder and a Post Graduate Certificate in Asperger Syndrome. She works part time with adults with autism and has written a number of books on ways to support, understand and appreciate people with conditions on the Autism Spectrum.

ISBN 9781847161642

£9.99